Copyright   ©201
WILMOORE   MD
All rights reserved. No part of this publication may be reproduced, distributed, or transmitted in any form or by any means, including photocopying, recording, or other electronic or mechanical methods, without the prior written permission of the publisher, except in the case of brief quotations embodied in critical reviews and certain other noncommercial uses permitted by copyright law.

Contents

INTRODUCTION 4
Mediterranean diet 6
    Plant based, not meat based 8
    Healthy fats 9
    What about wine 10
    Eating the Mediterranean way 10
    Fast facts about the Mediterranean diet 12
    Diet 13
    Why the Mediterranean diet 16
    How It Works 16
    The Research So Far 18
    Potential Pitfalls 21
    The Basics 22
    Avoid These Unhealthy Foods 23
    Foods to Eat 24
    What to Drink 26
    A Mediterranean Sample Menu for 1 Week 26
    Healthy Mediterranean Snacks 29
    How to Follow the Diet at Restaurants 30
    A Simple Shopping List for The Diet 30
    How to make the change 32
    What to do about mercury in fish 34

Make mealtimes a social experience 35
Start With These Recipes... 36
    Breakfast.. 38
    Salads and Sides.. 41
    Lunch and Dinner.. 44
Health Benefits of the Mediterranean Diet........................ 49
Mediterranean Diet And Weight loss.. 61
Focus on lifestyle changes 62
Consider calories without counting them 64
Eat more to lose weight. 65
Take portion size into account. 65
Watch your fat calories. 66
Increase the activity you love. 66
Suppress your appetite.. 67
Turn on your fullness hormones. 67
Control food cravings 68
Avoid blood sugar spikes. 68
Manage your stress hormones. 69
Tips on Loosing Weight on Mediteranean Diet..................... 70

INTRODUCTION

The Mediterranean diet has a long-standing reputation as one of the healthiest eating patterns around. It's also considered one of the most popular plans among dieters because it's flexible, rich in flavorful foods, and brimming with health benefits. In fact, the Mediterranean diet has been linked to increased weight loss, decreased inflammation, and a lower risk of chronic disease.

This book takes a look at the Mediterranean diet, including its benefits, potential drawbacks, foods to eat and avoid, and a sample meal plan.

The Mediterranean diet emphasizes mostly nutrient-rich, whole food ingredients like fruits, vegetables, healthy fats, and whole grains. Though it focuses primarily on plant foods, other ingredients like poultry, seafood, eggs, and dairy can also be enjoyed in moderation.

Meanwhile, processed foods, added sugars, refined grains, and sugar-sweetened beverages should be avoided. Certain types of alcohol, like red wine, can also be included in moderation but should be limited to no more than one or two servings per day for women and men, respectively.

In addition to making changes to your diet, engaging in regular physical activity is another crucial component of the Mediterranean diet. Walking, running, bicycling, rowing, playing sports, and lifting weights are just a few examples of healthy physical activities that you can add to your routine. Delicious food that's stood the test of time and helps keep you healthy for years to come. That's at the heart of the traditional Mediterranean diet.

There's no single Mediterranean diet plan, but in general, you'd be eating lots of fruits and vegetables, beans and nuts, healthy grains, fish, olive oil, small amounts of meat and dairy, and red wine. This lifestyle also encourages daily exercise, sharing meals with others, and enjoying it all.

Mediterranean diet

The Mediterranean diet is a modern nutritional model inspired by the traditional dietary patterns of some of the countries of the Mediterranean basin, particularly Southern Italy, Greece, Cyprus, Portugal, Turkey and Spain. Common to the diets of these regions are a high consumption of fruit and vegetables, bread and other cereals, olive oil and fish; making them low in saturated fat and high in monounsaturated fat and dietary fiber. A main factor in the appeal of the Mediterranean Diet is its rich, full flavored foods. Margarine and other unhealthy hydrogenated oils are considered bland and lacking the flavor olive oil can impart to foods.

Red wine is also consumed regularly but in moderate quantities. Chances are you have heard of the Mediterranean diet. If you have a chronic condition like heart disease or high blood pressure, your doctor may even have prescribed it to you. It is often promoted to decrease the risk of heart disease, depression, and dementia.

The traditional diets of countries bordering the Mediterranean Sea differ slightly so there are different versions of the Mediterranean diet. However, in 1993 the Harvard School of Public Health, Oldways Preservation and Exchange Trust, and the European Office of the World Health Organization introduced the Mediterranean Diet Pyramid as a guide to help familiarize people with the most common foods of the region. More of an eating pattern than a strictly regimented diet plan, the pyramid emphasized certain foods based on the dietary traditions of Crete, Greece, and southern Italy during the mid-20th century. At that time, these countries displayed low rates of chronic disease and higher than average adult life expectancy despite having limited access to healthcare. It was believed that the diet mainly fruits and vegetables, beans, nuts, whole grains, ûsh, olive oil, small amounts of dairy, and red wine contributed to their health benefits. The pyramid also highlighted daily exercise and the beneficial social aspects of eating meals together.

The Mediterranean diet is a way of eating based on the traditional cuisine of countries bordering the

Mediterranean Sea. While there is no single definition of the Mediterranean diet, it is typically high in vegetables, fruits, whole grains, beans, nut and seeds, and olive oil. The main components of Mediterranean diet include:

- Daily consumption of vegetables, fruits, whole grains and healthy fats
- Weekly intake of fish, poultry, beans and eggs
- Moderate portions of dairy products
- Limited intake of red meat

Other important elements of the Mediterranean diet are sharing meals with family and friends, enjoying a glass of red wine and being physically active.

Plant based, not meat based

The foundation of the Mediterranean diet is vegetables, fruits, herbs, nuts, beans and whole grains. Meals are built around these plant-based foods. Moderate amounts of dairy, poultry and eggs are also central to the

Mediterranean Diet, as is seafood. In contrast, red meat is eaten only occasionally.

Healthy fats

Healthy fats are a mainstay of the Mediterranean diet. They're eaten instead of less healthy fats, such as saturated and trans fats, which contribute to heart disease.

Olive oil is the primary source of added fat in the Mediterranean diet. Olive oil provides monounsaturated fat, which has been found to lower total cholesterol and low-density lipoprotein (LDL or "bad") cholesterol levels. Nuts and seeds also contain monounsaturated fat.

Fish are also important in the Mediterranean diet. Fatty fish such as mackerel, herring, sardines, albacore tuna, salmon and lake trout are rich in omega-3 fatty acids, a type of polyunsaturated fat that may reduce inflammation in the body. Omega-3 fatty acids also help decrease triglycerides, reduce blood clotting, and decrease the risk of stroke and heart failure.

What about wine

The Mediterranean diet typically allows red wine in moderation. Although alcohol has been associated with a reduced risk of heart disease in some studies, it's by no means risk free. The Dietary Guidelines for Americans caution against beginning to drink or drinking more often on the basis of potential health benefits.

Eating the Mediterranean way

Interested in trying the Mediterranean diet. These tips will help you get started:

- Eat more fruits and vegetables. Aim for 7 to 10 servings a day of fruit and vegetables.
- Opt for whole grains. Switch to whole-grain bread, cereal and pasta. Experiment with other whole grains, such as bulgur and farro.
- Use healthy fats. Try olive oil as a replacement for butter when cooking. Instead of putting butter or margarine on bread, try dipping it in flavored olive oil.

- Eat more seafood. Eat fish twice a week. Fresh or water-packed tuna, salmon, trout, mackerel and herring are healthy choices. Grilled fish tastes good and requires little cleanup. Avoid deep-fried fish.
- Reduce red meat. Substitute fish, poultry or beans for meat. If you eat meat, make sure it's lean and keep portions small.
- Enjoy some dairy. Eat low-fat Greek or plain yogurt and small amounts of a variety of cheeses.
- Spice it up. Herbs and spices boost flavor and lessen the need for salt.

The Mediterranean diet is a delicious and healthy way to eat. Many people who switch to this style of eating say they'll never eat any other way.

Fast facts about the Mediterranean diet

- There is no one Mediterranean diet. It consists of foods from a number of countries and regions including Spain, Greece, and Italy.
- The Mediterranean diet is a great way to replace the saturated fats in the average American diet.
- There is an emphasis on fruits, vegetables, lean meats, and natural sources.
- It is linked to good heart health, protection against diseases such as stroke, and prevention of diabetes.
- Moderation is still advised, as the diet has a high fat content.
- The Mediterranean diet should be paired with an active lifestyle for the best results.

Diet

The Mediterranean diet is a way to ensure food comes from a range of natural, healthful sources. The Mediterranean diet consists of:

- high quantities of vegetables, such as tomatoes, kale, broccoli, spinach, carrots, cucumbers, and onions
- fresh fruit such as apples, bananas, figs, dates, grapes, and melons.
- high consumption of legumes, beans, nuts, and seeds, such as almonds, walnuts, sunflower seeds, and cashews
- whole grains such as whole wheat, oats, barley, buckwheat, corn, and brown rice
- olive oil as the main source of dietary fat, alongside olives, avocados, and avocado oil
- cheese and yogurt as the main dairy foods, including Greek yogurt
- moderate amounts of fish and poultry, such as chicken, duck, turkey, salmon, sardines, and oysters

- eggs, including chicken, quail, and duck eggs
- limited amounts red meats and sweets
- around one glass per day of wine, with water as the main beverage of choice and no carbonated and sweetened drinks

This focus on plant foods and natural sources means that the Mediterranean diet contains nutrients such as:

- Healthful fats: The Mediterranean diet is known to be low in saturated fat and high in monounsaturated fat. Dietary guidelines for the United States recommend that saturated fat should make up no more than 10 percentTrusted Source of calorie intake.

- Fiber: The diet is high in fiber, which promotes healthy digestion and is believed to reduce the risk of bowel cancer and cardiovascular disease.

- High vitamin and mineral content: Fruits and vegetables provide vital vitamins and minerals, which regulate bodily processes. In addition, the presence of lean meats provides vitamins such as B-12 that are not found in plant foods.

- Low sugar: The diet is high in natural rather than added sugar, for example, in fresh fruits. Added sugar increases calories without nutritional benefit, is linked to diabetes and high blood pressure, and occurs in many of the processed foods absent from the Mediterranean diet. It is difficult to give exact nutritional information on the Mediterranean diet, since there is no single Mediterranean diet. This is because a variety of cultures and regions is involved.

Why the Mediterranean diet

Interest in the Mediterranean diet began in the 1960s with the observation that coronary heart disease caused fewer deaths in Mediterranean countries, such as Greece and Italy, than in the U.S. and northern Europe. Subsequent studies found that the Mediterranean diet is associated with reduced risk factors for cardiovascular disease.

The Mediterranean diet is one of the healthy eating plans recommended by the Dietary Guidelines for Americans to promote health and prevent chronic disease. It is also recognized by the World Health Organization as a healthy and sustainable dietary pattern and as an intangible cultural asset by the United National Educational, Scientific and Cultural Organization.

How It Works

The Mediterranean diet is a primarily plant-based eating plan that includes daily intake of whole grains, olive oil, fruits, vegetables, beans and other legumes, nuts, herbs, and spices. Other foods like animal proteins are eaten in smaller quantities, with the preferred animal protein being fish and seafood. Although the pyramid shape suggests the proportion of foods to eat (e.g., eat more fruits and vegetables and less dairy foods), it does not specify portion sizes or specific amounts. It is up to the individual to decide exactly how much food to eat at each meal, as this will vary by physical activity and body size. There are additional points that make this eating plan unique:

- An emphasis on healthy fats. Olive oil is recommended as the primary added fat, replacing other oils and fats (butter, margarine). Other foods naturally containing healthful fats are highlighted, such as avocados, nuts, and oily fish like salmon and sardines; among these, walnuts and fish are high in omega-3 fatty acids.
- Choosing fish as the preferred animal protein at least twice weekly and other animal proteins of poultry, eggs, and dairy (cheese or yogurt) in smaller portions either daily or a few times a week. Red meat is limited to a few times per month.

- Choosing water as the main daily beverage, but allowing a moderate intake of wine with meals, about one to two glasses a day for men and one glass a day for women.
- Stressing daily physical activity through enjoyable activities.

The Research So Far

Research has consistently shown that the Mediterranean diet is effective in reducing the risk of cardiovascular diseases and overall mortality. A study of nearly 26,000 women found that those who followed this type of diet had 25% less risk of developing cardiovascular disease over the course of 12 years. The study examined a range of underlying mechanisms that might account for this reduction, and found that changes in inflammation, blood sugar, and body mass index were the biggest drivers.

One interesting finding of this eating plan is that it dispels the myth that people with or at risk for heart disease must eat a low fat diet. Although it does matter which types of fats are chosen, the percentage of calories from fat is less of an issue. A primary prevention trial including thousands of people with diabetes or other risk factors for heart disease found that a Mediterranean diet supplemented with extra virgin olive oil or nuts and without any fat and calorie restrictions reduced the rates of death from stroke by roughly 30%. Most dietary fats were healthy fats, such as those from fatty fish, olive oil, and nuts, but total fat intake was generous at 39-42% of total daily calories, much higher than the 20-35% fat guideline as stated by the Institute of Medicine.

There has also been increased interest in the diet s effects on aging and cognitive function. Cell damage through stress and inflammation that can lead to age-related diseases has been linked to a specific part of DNA called telomeres. These structures naturally shorten with age, and their length size can predict life expectancy and the risk of developing age-related diseases. Telomeres with long lengths are considered protective against chronic diseases and earlier death, whereas short lengths increase risk. Antioxidants can help combat cell stress and preserve telomere length, such as by eating foods that contain antioxidants nutrients like fruits, vegetables, nuts, and whole grains. These foods are found in healthy eating patterns like the Mediterranean diet. This was demonstrated in a large cohort of 4676 healthy middle-aged women from the Nurses Health Study where participants who more closely followed the Mediterranean diet were found to have longer telomere length.

Another Nurses Health Study following 10,670 women ages 57-61 observed the effect of dietary patterns on aging. Healthy aging was defined as living to 70 years or more, and having no chronic diseases (e.g., type 2 diabetes, kidney disease, lung disease, Parkinson s disease, cancer) or major declines in mental health, cognition, and physical function. The study found that the women who followed a Mediterranean-type eating pattern were 46% more likely to age healthfully. Increased intake of plant foods, whole grains, and fish; moderate alcohol intake; and low intake of red and processed meats were believed to contribute to this finding.

Potential Pitfalls

There is a risk of excess calorie intake because specific amounts of foods and portion sizes are not emphasized, which could lead to weight gain. It might be helpful to use the Mediterranean Diet Pyramid, which provides guidance on specific types of foods to choose, along with a balanced plate guide such as the Harvard Healthy Eating Plate, which gives a better indication of proportions of food to eat per meal. However, it is important to note that probably in part due to the higher intake of olive oil and less processed foods the Mediterranean dietary pattern provides satiety and enables long term adherence. In one of the most successful weight loss trials to date, those assigned to the Mediterranean diet maintained weight loss over a period of six years.

Research supports the health benefits of a Mediterranean-style eating pattern that includes several different foods. It is the combination of these foods that appear protective against disease, as the benefit is not as strong when looking at single foods or nutrients included in the Mediterranean diet. Therefore it is important to not simply add olive oil or nuts to one s current diet but to adopt the plan in its entirety.

The Basics

- Eat: Vegetables, fruits, nuts, seeds, legumes, potatoes, whole grains, breads, herbs, spices, fish, seafood and extra virgin olive oil.
- Eat in moderation: Poultry, eggs, cheese and yogurt.
- Eat only rarely: Red meat.
- Don't eat: Sugar-sweetened beverages, added sugars, processed meat, refined grains, refined oils and other highly processed foods.

Avoid These Unhealthy Foods

You should avoid these unhealthy foods and ingredients:

- Added sugar: Soda, candies, ice cream, table sugar and many others.
- Refined grains: White bread, pasta made with refined wheat, etc.
- Trans fats: Found in margarine and various processed foods.
- Refined oils: Soybean oil, canola oil, cottonseed oil and others.
- Processed meat: Processed sausages, hot dogs, etc.

Highly processed foods: Anything labeled "low-fat" or "diet" or which looks like it was made in a factory. You must read food labels carefully if you want to avoid these unhealthy ingredients.

Foods to Eat

Exactly which foods belong to the Mediterranean diet is controversial, partly because there is such variation between different countries. The diet examined by most studies is high in healthy plant foods and relatively low in animal foods.

However, eating fish and seafood is recommended at least twice a week. The Mediterranean lifestyle also involves regular physical activity, sharing meals with other people and enjoying life. You should base your diet on these healthy, unprocessed Mediterranean foods:

- Vegetables: Tomatoes, broccoli, kale, spinach, onions, cauliflower, carrots, Brussels sprouts, cucumbers, etc.
- Fruits: Apples, bananas, oranges, pears, strawberries, grapes, dates, figs, melons, peaches, etc.
- Nuts and seeds: Almonds, walnuts, macadamia nuts, hazelnuts, cashews, sunflower seeds, pumpkin seeds, etc.

- Legumes: Beans, peas, lentils, pulses, peanuts, chickpeas, etc.
- Tubers: Potatoes, sweet potatoes, turnips, yams, etc.
- Whole grains: Whole oats, brown rice, rye, barley, corn, buckwheat, whole wheat, whole-grain bread and pasta.
- Fish and seafood: Salmon, sardines, trout, tuna, mackerel, shrimp, oysters, clams, crab, mussels, etc.
- Poultry: Chicken, duck, turkey, etc.
- Eggs: Chicken, quail and duck eggs.
- Dairy: Cheese, yogurt, Greek yogurt, etc.
- Herbs and spices: Garlic, basil, mint, rosemary, sage, nutmeg, cinnamon, pepper, etc.
- Healthy Fats: Extra virgin olive oil, olives, avocados and avocado oil.

Whole, single-ingredient foods are the key to good health.

What to Drink

Water should be your go-to beverage on a Mediterranean diet.

This diet also includes moderate amounts of red wine around 1 glass per day. However, this is completely optional, and wine should be avoided by anyone with alcoholism or problems controlling their consumption.

Coffee and tea are also completely acceptable, but you should avoid sugar-sweetened beverages and fruit juices, which are very high in sugar.

A Mediterranean Sample Menu for 1 Week

Below is a sample menu for one week on the Mediterranean diet. Feel free to adjust the portions and food choices based on your own needs and preferences.

Monday

- Breakfast: Greek yogurt with strawberries and oats.
- Lunch: Whole-grain sandwich with vegetables.

- Dinner: A tuna salad, dressed in olive oil. A piece of fruit for dessert.

Tuesday

- Breakfast: Oatmeal with raisins.
- Lunch: Leftover tuna salad from the night before.
- Dinner: Salad with tomatoes, olives and feta cheese.

Wednesday

- Breakfast: Omelet with veggies, tomatoes and onions. A piece of fruit.
- Lunch: Whole-grain sandwich, with cheese and fresh vegetables.
- Dinner: Mediterranean lasagne.

Thursday

- Breakfast: Yogurt with sliced fruits and nuts.
- Lunch: Leftover lasagne from the night before.
- Dinner: Broiled salmon, served with brown rice and vegetables.

Friday

- Breakfast: Eggs and vegetables, fried in olive oil.
- Lunch: Greek yogurt with strawberries, oats and nuts.
- Dinner: Grilled lamb, with salad and baked potato.

Saturday

- Breakfast: Oatmeal with raisins, nuts and an apple.
- Lunch: Whole-grain sandwich with vegetables.
- Dinner: Mediterranean pizza made with whole wheat, topped with cheese, vegetables and olives.

Sunday

- Breakfast: Omelet with veggies and olives.
- Lunch: Leftover pizza from the night before.
- Dinner: Grilled chicken, with vegetables and a potato. Fruit for dessert.

There is usually no need to count calories or track macronutrients (protein, fat and carbs) on the Mediterranean diet.

Healthy Mediterranean Snacks

You don't need to eat more than 3 meals per day. But if you become hungry between meals, there are plenty of healthy snack options:

- A handful of nuts.
- A piece of fruit.
- Carrots or baby carrots.
- Some berries or grapes.
- Leftovers from the night before.
- Greek yogurt.

- Apple slices with almond butter.

How to Follow the Diet at Restaurants

Its very simple to make most restaurant meals suitable for the Mediterranean diet.

- Choose fish or seafood as your main dish.
- Ask them to fry your food in extra virgin olive oil.
- Only eat whole-grain bread, with olive oil instead of butter.

A Simple Shopping List for The Diet

It is always a good idea to shop at the perimeter of the store. That's usually where the whole foods are. Always try to choose the least-processed option. Organic is best, but only if you can easily afford it.

- Vegetables: Carrots, onions, broccoli, spinach, kale, garlic, etc.
- Fruits: Apples, bananas, oranges, grapes, etc.
- Berries: Strawberries, blueberries, etc.

- Frozen veggies: Choose mixes with healthy vegetables.
- Grains: Whole-grain bread, whole-grain pasta, etc.
- Legumes: Lentils, pulses, beans, etc.
- Nuts: Almonds, walnuts, cashews, etc.
- Seeds: Sunflower seeds, pumpkin seeds, etc.
- Condiments: Sea salt, pepper, turmeric, cinnamon, etc.
- Fish: Salmon, sardines, mackerel, trout.
- Shrimp and shellfish.
- Potatoes and sweet potatoes.
- Cheese.
- Greek yogurt.
- Chicken.
- Pastured or omega-3 enriched eggs.
- Olives.
- Extra virgin olive oil.

It is best to clear all unhealthy temptations from your home, including sodas, ice cream, candy, pastries, white bread, crackers and processed foods. If you only have healthy food in your home, you will eat healthy food.

Though there is not one defined Mediterranean diet, this way of eating is generally rich in healthy plant foods and relatively lower in animal foods, with a focus on fish and seafood.

You can find a whole world of information about the Mediterranean diet on the internet, and many great books have been written about it. At the end of the day, the Mediterranean diet is incredibly healthy and satisfying. You won't be disappointed.

How to make the change

If you re feeling daunted by the thought of changing your eating habits to a Mediterranean diet, here are some suggestions to get you started:

- Eat lots of vegetables. Try a simple plate of sliced tomatoes drizzled with olive oil and crumbled feta cheese, or load your thin crust pizza with peppers and mushrooms instead of sausage and pepperoni. Salads, soups, and crudité platters are also great ways to load up on vegetables.

- Always eat breakfast. Fruit, whole grains, and other fiber-rich foods are a great way to start your day, keeping you pleasantly full for hours.
- Eat seafood twice a week. Fish such as tuna, salmon, herring, sablefish (black cod), and sardines are rich in Omega-3 fatty acids, and shellfish like mussels, oysters, and clams have similar benefits for brain and heart health.
- Cook a vegetarian meal one night a week. If it s helpful, you can jump on the Meatless Mondays trend of foregoing meat on the first day of the week, or simply pick a day where you build meals around beans, whole grains, and vegetables. Once you get the hang of it, try two nights a week.
- Enjoy dairy products in moderation. The USDA recommends limiting saturated fat to no more than 10% of your daily calories (about 200 calories for most people). That still allows you to enjoy dairy

products such as natural (unprocessed) cheese, Greek or plain yogurt.
- For dessert, eat fresh fruit. Instead of ice cream, cake or other baked goods, opt for strawberries, fresh figs, grapes, or apples.
- Use good fats. Extra-virgin olive oil, nuts, sunflower seeds, olives, and avocados are great sources of healthy fats for your daily meals.

What to do about mercury in fish

Despite all the health benefits of seafood, nearly all fish and shellfish contain traces of pollutants, including the toxic metal mercury. These guidelines can help you make the safest choices.

The concentration of mercury and other pollutants increases in larger fish, so it s best to avoid eating large fish like shark, swordfish, tilefish, and king mackerel. Most adults can safely eat about 12 ounces (two 6-ounce servings) of other types of cooked seafood a week. Pay attention to local seafood advisories to learn if fish you ve caught is safe to eat.

For women who are pregnant, nursing mothers, and children aged 12 and younger, choose fish and shellfish that are lower in mercury, such as shrimp, canned light tuna, salmon, Pollock, or catfish. Because of its higher mercury content, eat no more than 6 ounces (one average meal) of albacore tuna per week.

Make mealtimes a social experience

The simple act of talking to a friend or loved over the dinner table can play a big role in relieving stress and boosting mood. Eating with others can also prevent overeating, making it as healthy for your waistline as it is for your outlook. Switch off the TV and computer, put away your smartphone, and connect to someone over a meal.

- Gather the family together and stay up to date with each other s daily lives. Regular family meals provide comfort to kids and are a great way to monitor their eating habits as well.

- Share meals with others to expand your social network. If you live alone, cook a little extra and invite a friend, coworker, or neighbor to join you.
- Cook with others. Invite a friend to share shopping and cooking responsibilities for a Mediterranean meal. Cooking with others can be a fun way to deepen relationships and splitting the costs can make it cheaper for both of you.

Start With These Recipes

People who follow the Mediterranean diet have a longer life expectancy and lower rates of chronic diseases than do other adults. Indeed, the Dietary Guidelines for Americans point to the Mediterranean diet as an example of a healthy-eating plan.

The Mediterranean diet emphasizes plant-based foods, such as fruits and vegetables, whole grains, legumes and nuts. It replaces butter with healthy fats, such as olive oil and canola oil, and uses herbs and spices instead of salt to flavor foods. Red meat is limited to no more than a few times a month, while fish should be on the menu twice a week. The Mediterranean diet is also about enjoying delicious foods as you'll discover when you try these recipes.

With no rigid rules around cutting out macronutrients but an emphasis on eating more heart-healthy foods, this particular diet is one of the most sustainable ones around. But our favorite part about it is that the kind of ingredients it prioritizes allows for some seriously good eating. With rich tahini sauce, fruity olive oil, nutty whole grains, plenty of fish and eggs, and tons of fresh herbs and spices all getting two thumbs up, just imagine the meals you can make.

But if you are still not sure where to begin or are simply overwhelmed by the options, here are 23 of our picks for the best and simplest Mediterranean diet recipes. Short of actually flying out to that sunny coastline, creating these dishes at home is the best way to kick off your new and improved lifestyle.

Breakfast
1. Mediterranean Vegetable Frittata

With bright red and green vegetables scattered throughout its eggy batter, this frittata is just as pretty as it is healthy. Fresh oregano leaves and crumbled feta add a touch of savory with a creamy consistency, making it a perfect warm meal to start off the day.

2. Greek Tofu Scramble

Honor the Mediterranean diet s emphasis on plant-based eating with this produce-packed, vegan protein-rich breakfast. It s bursting with veggies, but the tahini and nutritional yeast are the real heroes for adding a ton of rich flavor to the crumbled tofu.

3. Mediterranean-Flavored Overnight Oats

Overnight oats are all the rage, but even veteran nutrition nuts might be pleasantly surprised by this unique, Mediterranean-inspired concoction. With ricotta cheese, blood oranges, pistachios, and lavender honey (if you can find it), it s a fruity bowl that s just creamy enough to make you appreciate oats again.

4. Scrambled Eggs in Caramelized Onions and Paprika

You don t have to settle for plain old scrambled eggs when you re on the Mediterranean diet. The whipped eggs in this recipe are stirred into a mixture of caramelized onion, tomato, and lots of herbs. Add feta if you wish, but it s just as tasty if you choose to go dairy-free.

5. Orange and Almond Granola

Extra virgin olive oil may sound like an unusual ingredient for granola, but don t knock it til you try it. It s a seriously good complement to the honey and orange zest, and you re still getting plenty of nutty, crunchy substance from the almonds and baked oats.

6. Breakfast Tabbouleh

With bulgur, lots of parsley, and an olive oil and lemon dressing, this is pretty much your typical tabbouleh. But the addition of eggs gives it some much-needed protein that makes it all the more breakfasty. Poaching them will require five extra minutes, but when you ve got runny egg yolk to dip your pita wedges into, you ll be grateful you took that time.

7. Honey Lemon Ricotta Breakfast Toast With Figs and Pistachios

Give peanut butter a break and spread your toast with a layer of whipped ricotta lemon and honey instead. The lemon s tart and zesty flavor liven up the entire recipe, while sliced figs and pistachios on top get that sweet and savory combo just right.

8. Mediterranean Sweet Potato Hash

Sweet potatoes replace the white ones in this healthy hash, and while you won t find bacon in the mix, you won t even notice it s missing. This blogger changes things up by adding green olives and mozzarella balls, and let s not forget about the juicy pomegranate seeds that make the dish totally unique.

Salads and Sides
9. Mediterranean Cauliflower Salad

The Mediterranean diet doesnt have anything against carbs, per se (you can eat pasta), but for the times you do want to cut back, opt for this grain salad. Cauliflower has been pulverized and microwaved until tender, then tossed with a heap of other veggies and a ridiculously easy dressing. You ll feel like you re eating rice, but really it s veggies.

10. Fattoush

With bits of toasted pita, chopped vegetables, fresh herbs, and a lemon- and garlic-infused olive oil dressing, this traditional Lebanese bread salad is the ideal light lunch. Need some extra protein? Add chickpeas, feta, or grilled chicken to make it more filling.

11. Fresh Fava Bean Salad

Chickpeas usually take the spotlight when we think of Mediterranean food (hello, falafel and hummus), but don t forget, there are plenty of other legumes that are worth incorporating into your meals. This salad mixes fresh, protein-packed boiled fava beans with olive oil-flavored homemade croutons and lots of Kalamata olives for a lettuce-free salad you ll be eating by the forkful.

12. Yogurt Tahini Mediterranean Carrot Salad

The Mediterranean diet doesn t have much space for mayonnaise, but if it s a creamy carrot salad you re looking for, this one totally delivers. The tahini and Greek yogurt dressing offers much more healthy fat and protein than mayo, while feta and parsley amp up the Mediterranean vibe.

13. Spiced Chickpeas

Chickpeas are good for more than just hummus, guys! Combine them in a pan with cardamom, cumin, and some red pepper flakes, and they become spicy, crispy, and totally addictive. Toss them into salads or eat them on their own as a delicious side or snack.

14. Muhammara

You can always find hummus at the store, but one must-have dip that isn t so readily available at the supermarket is this traditional Syrian red pepper and walnut one. While there s usually a piece of bread blended into the mix for texture, this recipe opts for rolled oats. But otherwise, it keeps the cumin-spiced, garlicky flavors of the classic.

15. Greek Style Lemon Roasted Potatoes

You re hit with an intense craving for fries, but you re really trying to lay off the whole deep-fried thing. Make these oven-cooked potatoes instead. Coated in olive oil, garlic powder, and a hint of lemon juice, then roasted, they have the crispy outsides and buttery insides that are reminiscent of thick-cut wedges. We re pretty sure they ll hit the spot.

Lunch and Dinner
16. Mediterranean Chickpea Tuna Pitas

Chickpeas step in for chicken, and once again, tahini replaces mayo in the creamy sauce for this totally vegan take on the deli salad. And since we re going

Mediterranean, it s tucked into pita pockets instead of sliced bread, alongside basil, cherry tomatoes, and olives.

17. Mediterranean Sheet-Pan Salmon

If it s heart-healthy and Mediterranean-diet approved, so this sheet-pan salmon definitely makes the cut. The fish itself is a powerhouse of omega-3 fatty acids, but if that s not enough, the olive oil coating and pitted olive garnish make sure your system runs like a well-oiled machine.

18. Tomato and Roasted Mediterranean Vegetable Risotto

With the Mediterranean area including Italy, how could the cuisine not be super drool-worthy? And while the cheesy pizzas and rich pasta are more famous, this risotto reflects the region s pride in fresh produce. It s loaded with all sorts of vegetables in a tomato-based broth that doesn t involve any dairy whatsoever.

19. Mediterranean Turkey Burger

The Mediterranean diet isn t huge on red meat, so these turkey patties are a great way to satisfy a burger craving instead. Seasoned with oregano and parsley, they re especially tasty with a hefty drizzle of the Greek yogurt tzatziki sauce so much better than plain old ketchup and mustard.

20. Harissa Pasta

Although harissa is a spice paste from North Africa, it frequently makes an appearance in Mediterranean cooking, probably thanks to the geographic proximity of the regions. Whatever the reason, we re grateful because it makes this pasta possible.

21. Healthy Mediterranean Chicken Orzo

With oregano, basil, parsley, olives, and feta, this orzo is practically a hall of fame for Mediterranean cuisine s biggest stars. The fresh ingredients add flavor to the whole-wheat orzo and chicken, and if the taste alone isn t incentive enough to make it, maybe the fact that it s ready in fewer than 30 minutes will be!

22. Mediterranean Veggie Tacos

You can even give tacos the Mediterranean diet treatment by stuffing crunchy tortilla shells with ingredients like olives, feta, hummus, and Greek dressing. Not only are these a nice change to typical Taco Tuesday, but the no-cook method makes them even easier to whip up for a quick meal.

23. Cumin Beef Fried Rice

Fried rice isn t just a Chinese take-out dish. This recipe takes a more Mediterranean route, using cumin and sumac, a lemony spice common in the region s cuisine, to season the meat, egg, and grains. It s a well-balanced, nourishing meal, all ready in one pan and 30 minutes.

Health Benefits of the Mediterranean Diet

The Mediterranean diet is not specifically a weight loss diet, but cutting out red meats, animal fats, and processed food may lead to weight loss.

In areas where the diet is consumed, there are lower rates of mortality and heart disease, and other benefits.

Eating this diet, which is rich in fruits and vegetables, healthy fats, and whole grains, can lower your risk for certain health problems. Here are a few ways you can improve your health by eating the Mediterranean Diet.

Out of all the trendy diets you could choose, following a Mediterranean diet is not only delicious (and may make you feel like you re on vacay in Greece), it could boost your health. Packed with fruits and veggies, fish, whole grains, and healthful fats, the Mediterranean diet could help manage your weight, benefit your brain, improve heart health, and maybe even help you live longer. Watch the video above or scroll down to learn about the seven ways you can improve your health by eating a Mediterranean Diet.

1. The Mediterranean Diet May Help Reduce Your Risk for Heart Disease

Numerous studies suggest the Mediterranean diet is good for your ticker, noted a meta-analysis published in November 2015 in the journal Critical Reviews in Food Science and Nutrition. Perhaps the most convincing evidence comes from a randomized clinical trial published in April 2013 in the New England Journal of Medicine. For about five years, authors followed 7,000 women and men in Spain who had type 2 diabetes or a high risk for cardiovascular disease. Those who ate a calorie-unrestricted Mediterranean diet with extra-virgin olive oil or nuts had a 30 percent lower risk of heart events. Researchers didnt advise participants on exercise.

The study authors reanalyzed the data at a later point to address a widely criticized flaw in the randomization protocol, and reported similar results in June 2018 in the New England Journal of Medicine. That is probably the biggest scientific evidence to say that a Mediterranean diet is healthful, in terms of reducing the risk of cardiovascular.

2. Eating a Mediterranean Diet May Reduce Women s Risk for Stroke

We already know from the PREDIMED study that eating in a Mediterranean fashion can help lower the risk of cardiovascular disease in some people. Well, the diet may also help reduce stroke risk in women, though researchers didn t observe the same results in men.

Researchers looked at a predominantly white group of 23,232 men and women ages 40 to 77 who lived in the United Kingdom. The more closely a woman followed a Mediterranean diet, the lower her risk of having a stroke. However, researchers didnt see statistically significant results in men. Most notably, in women who were at high risk of having a stroke, following the diet reduced their chances of this health event by 20 percent.

Study authors don t know the reason for the difference, but they hypothesize that different types of strokes in men and women may play a role. A good next step toward understanding the reasons behind the differences would be a clinical trial.

3. A Mediterranean Diet May Prevent Cognitive Decline and Alzheimer s Disease

As a heart-healthy diet, the Mediterranean eating pattern may also help to reduce a decline in your memory and thinking skills with age. The brain is a very hungry organ. To supply all of those nutrients and oxygen [that it needs], you have to have a rich blood supply. So, people who are having any problems with their vascular health   their blood vessels   are really at increased risk for developing problems with their brain, and then that frequently will present itself as cognitive decline.

A July 2016 review published in the journal Frontiers in Nutrition looked at the effect of the Mediterranean diet on cognitive function and concluded there is encouraging evidence that a higher adherence to a Mediterranean diet is associated with improving cognition, slowing cognitive decline, or reducing the conversion to Alzheimer s disease.

Whats more, a small study funded by the National Institute on Aging and published in May 2018 in the journal Neurology looked at brain scans for 70 people who had no signs of dementia at the outset, and scored them for how closely their eating patterns hewed to the Mediterranean pattern. (8) Those who scored low tended to have more beta-amyloid deposits (protein plaques in the brain associated with Alzheimer s disease) and lower energy use in the brain at the end of the study. At least two years later, these individuals also showed a greater increase of deposits and reduction of energy use potentially signaling an increased risk for Alzheimer is than those who more closely followed the Mediterranean diet.

All that said, more research is needed before recommending this eating approach to lower Alzheimer s risk. The authors called for additional research in a larger participant group and for a longer study period.

For now, Dr. Fargo identifies the Mediterranean diet as one way of eating that can help stave off cognitive decline. But he does not necessarily recommend it over other well-studied diets, such as the MIND diet (MIND stands for Mediterranean DASH Diet Intervention for Neurodegenerative Delay), which is a hybrid of the Mediterranean pattern and the blood-pressure lowering DASH diet, noted an article published in September 2015 in the journal Alzheimer's and Dementia. What the Alzheimers Association recommends is a heart-healthy pattern of eating. Also urges caution in drawing conclusions about the current body of research into how diets affect the development of Alzheimer s disease, saying that the exact mechanisms at play are still unclear.

4. The Mediterranean Diet May Help With Weight Loss and Maintenance

Likely due to its focus on whole, fresh foods, the Mediterranean diet may help you lose weight in a safe and sustainable way, but if you re looking for fast results, you may be better off with a different diet plan. As mentioned, in its 2019 rankings, U.S. News & World Report rated the Mediterranean diet as No. 1 in its Best Diets Overall category, yet the diet tied with several other plans for the 17th position among the website s Best Weight Loss Diets. Over a five-year period, eating a calorie-unrestricted Mediterranean diet high in unsaturated vegetable fat led to slightly more weight loss and added less to participants waist circumferences than a low-fat diet, according to an analysis of the Spanish PREDIMED trial data that was published in August 2016 in the journal The Lancet: Diabetes and Endocrinology. Particularly, people who added extra-virgin olive oil to their diets lost the most weight 0.88 kilograms (kg), or 1.9 pounds (lbs) on average. Those who added nuts lost 0.4 kg on average

(0.88 lbs), and those in the control group who ate a low-fat diet lost 0.6 kg (1.3 lbs).

Once you add calorie restriction, the Mediterranean diet may show more dramatic results, though not necessarily beating out another popular diet approach. In a two-year randomized, clinical trial, 322 moderately obese middle-aged participants in Israel, who were mostly men, followed one of three diets: a calorie-restricted low-fat diet, a calorie-restricted Mediterranean diet, and a calorie-unrestricted low-carb diet.

Among the Mediterranean diet followers, women ate a maximum of 1,500 calories per day, while men s calorie count was restricted to 1,800 calories per day, with the goal of having no more than 35 percent of their calories from fat. The calorie restrictions were the same for those on the low-fat diet. The mean weight loss was 4.4 kg (9.7 lbs) for the Mediterranean-diet group, 2.9 kg (6.4 lbs) for the low-fat group, and 4.7 kg (10.3 lbs) for the low-carbohydrate group.

5. Eating a Mediterranean Diet May Help Stave Off and Manage Type 2 Diabetes

For type 2 diabetes management and possible prevention, a Mediterranean diet may be the way to go. Using participants from the PREDIMED study, researchers randomized a subgroup of 418 people ages 55 to 80 without diabetes and followed up with them after four years to see if they had developed the disease. The results were published in the journal Diabetes Care. Those participants who followed the Mediterranean diet, whether supplementing with olive oil or nuts, had a 52 percent lower risk for type 2 diabetes during the four year follow-up, and they didn t necessarily lose weight or exercise more.

Furthermore, a meta-analysis of 20 randomized clinical trials published in January 2013 in the American Journal of Clinical Nutrition found that the Mediterranean diet improved blood sugar control more than low-carbohydrate, low-glycemic index, and high-protein diets, in those managing type 2 diabetes. This finding suggests that a Mediterranean diet may be an effective way to help ward off type 2 diabetes related health complications.

6. People With Rheumatoid Arthritis May Benefit From the Mediterranean Diet

Rheumatoid arthritis (RA) is an autoimmune disease in which the body s immune system mistakenly attacks the joints, creating pain and swelling in and around them. Certain properties of the Mediterranean diet, including its richness in anti-inflammatory omega-3 fatty acids, may help relieve RA symptoms.

According to the National Institutes of Health's Office of Dietary Supplements, research thus far suggests that long-chain omega-3 fatty acids (found in fatty fish) may be helpful in relieving RA symptoms on top of medication, though more research is needed.

7. Are Foods in the Mediterranean Diet Protective Against Cancer

Indeed, a Mediterranean diet meal plan may help prevent certain types of cancer. A meta-analysis and review of 83 studies published in October 2017 in the journal Nutrients suggested the Mediterranean diet may help reduce the risk of cancers such as breast cancer and colorectal cancer, and help prevent cancer-related death. These observed beneficial effects are mainly driven by higher intakes of fruits, vegetables, and whole grains.

A separate study, published in October 2015 in the journal JAMA Internal Medicine and based on PREDIMED data, found that women who ate a Mediterranean diet supplemented with extra-virgin olive oil had a 62 percent lower risk of breast cancer than those in the control group that ate a low-fat diet.

8. Eating Foods in a Mediterranean Diet May Help Ease Depression

The Mediterranean way of eating is linked to lower incidence of depression, according to an analysis of 41 observational studies published in September 2018 in the journal Molecular Psychiatry. Analysis of pooled data from four longitudinal studies revealed that the diet was associated with a 33 percent reduced risk of depression, compared with following a pro-inflammatory diet (richer in processed meats, sugar, and trans fats) that is more typical of a standard American diet.

While the study didn t reveal why a Mediterranean diet lowered depression risk, the study authors wrote that their results may be a launching point to develop and study diet-based interventions for depression.

Mediterranean Diet And Weight loss

Weight loss is an important issue for many people (and perhaps you) in the world today. You may be looking for a way to lose some weight and think that the Mediterranean diet is the way to go. Choosing a Mediterranean diet isn't going to be a traditional "diet" or a quick fix.

Rather, it's a series of healthy lifestyle choices that can get you to your weight loss goal while you eat delicious, flavorful foods and get out and enjoy life. Sounds much better than counting calories and depriving yourself, right?

With that description in mind, you need to focus on a few must-haves with the Mediterranean lifestyle in order to lose weight successfully. You have to pay attention to lifestyle changes, manage your calorie intake through balancing food choices and controlling portions, and increase your physical activity.

Focus on lifestyle changes

The focus of the Mediterranean diet is on your entire lifestyle. Paying attention to lifestyle changes, such as changing your portion sizes and exercising regularly, is the only way to see long-term results. Weight-loss diets come and go, and most can help you lose the weight, but they aren't something you can live with long term.

The Mediterranean diet helps you pay attention to your individual lifestyle, including the types of foods you eat, the portion sizes you consume, your physical activities, and your overall way of life. You can incorporate these changes into your daily life and create long-term habits that bring you not only weight loss but also sustained weight loss.

- Set realistic, practical, and measurable goals
- Quit diets once and for all.
- Make time in a fast-paced lifestyle.
- When incorporating the Mediterranean diet into your lifestyle, your first goal is to try to slow down. Look at all you have on your (figurative)

plate and see whether you can start to say "no" to some things so you can free up time for yourself.
- Create small changes that stick.
- Look at small goals you can integrate into your daily life and do it.

Consider calories without counting them

Calories are one of the most important concepts of weight loss. Basically, calories are the amount of energy in the foods you eat and the amount of energy your body uses for daily activities. Your body constantly needs energy or fuel not only for daily activities such as cooking, cleaning, and exercising but also for basic biological functions (like, you know, breathing).

Everyone has a different metabolic rate that determines how quickly he or she burns calories and depends on factors such as age, genetics, gender, and physical fitness level.

At the end of the day, you can't lose weight if you eat more calories than you burn through daily activity and exercise. To lose weight, you have to create a calorie deficit, but you can do so without actually knowing how many calories you burn. All you have to do is make small changes to your lifestyle, such as reducing portion sizes and exercising more, to reduce your calorie intake.

Eat more to lose weight.

Unlike many weight-loss diets, a Mediterranean style of eating lets you have more food on your plate while still taking in fewer calories. Eat far more low-calorie vegetables and fewer high-calorie meats and grains. As an added bonus, these lower-calorie foods also help you feel more satisfied with your meal instead of feeling deprived.

Take portion size into account.

Paying attention to portion sizes is a far better way to decrease your calorie intake than counting calories. Portion sizes in the Mediterranean are different than they are in the United States, which is one reason folks in the Mediterranean region tend to manage their weights more effectively.

Watch your fat calories.

The Mediterranean diet also allows you to keep track of the calories you get from fat. Although people on the Mediterranean coast eat slightly more fat than is recommended in the United States (35 percent of their calories come from fat, versus the U.S. recommendation of 30 percent), they consume different types of fat, such as the healthy fats from olive oil.

Increase the activity you love.

Exercise is an important component to weight loss and health, especially with the Mediterranean diet. You have to use up some of your calorie intake as energy, or those calories will store as fat. Exercise allows you to not only burn calories but also strengthen your heart, manage stress, and increase your energy level.

Suppress your appetite

Eating a Mediterranean style diet is not only great for your health but can also work as a natural appetite suppressant to help manage your weight. When you eat the right balance of plant-based foods and healthy fats, your body works in a natural way to feel satisfied. Because you're full, you're not tempted (at least, not by your stomach) to snack on high-calorie junk food a short while after your last meal.

Turn on your fullness hormones.

The Mediterranean diet is naturally high in low-glycemic foods, those carbohydrate-containing foods that illicit a lower blood sugar spike. Low-glycemic foods may just help kick on your fullness response. Appetite is controlled by an intricate dance of hormones that trigger the feelings of hunger and fullness.

Control food cravings

Food cravings occur for many reasons, whether they're physiological, psychological, or a combination of both. For instance, having a stressful day at work may lead to food cravings. Unfortunately, no one-size-fits-all-answer exists to deal with food cravings, but you can do a few things to manage them more effectively.

Avoid blood sugar spikes.

Make sure you don't skip meals or wait longer than 5 hours to eat. Eat a meal or snack every 3 to 5 hours. Eat when you are hungry instead of waiting until you have extreme hunger.

Eat protein-rich foods and a bit of fat. Include foods such as fish, beans, nuts, or eggs with a fat with each meal to help slow down your digestion

Eat high-fiber, fruits, vegetables, grains, and legumes with each meal and snack. You don't have to eat these foods all at once, but including some combination of them at meals and incorporating a fruit, veggie, or whole grain with your snacks is a good idea.

Manage your stress hormones.

You can accomplish this by exercising, getting enough sleep, drinking water, practicing deep breathing, meditating, and relaxing. For example, if you are getting ready for a stressful meeting, take a few moments to do some deep breathing. Simply take a deep breath, hold it for a few seconds, and let the air out. Keep repeating for as long as you can. Even a few minutes can help.

Tips on Loosing Weight on Mediteranean Diet

You can lose weight on the Mediterranean Diet. New research coming from the now known PREDIMED study, a long-term nutritional intervention study aimed to assess the efficacy of the Mediterranean diet in the primary prevention of cardiovascular diseases, showed that people lost slightly more weight when following a Mediterranean diet, compared to a low-fat diet. They also had the least increase in waist circumference compared to the low-fat diet. Of course this is not the first time the Mediterranean diet has been associated with weight loss, another study in 2008 published in the New England Journal of Medicine also showed that there was greater weight loss with the Mediterranean diet compared to a low-fat diet. Other studies have also associated the Mediterranean diet with a healthy weight in children as well as in pregnant women.

So it is not something new. Now, to clarify, many people associate the Mediterranean diet with lots of pasta and olive oil. That is a misconception, the traditional

Mediterranean diet that had as a prototype the Cretan diet is mainly plants and olive oil with some carbs interspersed, it is a moderate to high fat diet with a moderate amount of carbohydrates. If you want to lose weight following a Mediterranean diet here are my tips that work.

1. Eat your main meal early in the day

Traditionally within a Mediterranean diet, lunch is the main meal , it being consumed between 1 to 3 pm. By moving a larger meal early in the day, you reduce the risk of overeating later. In fact a Spanish study showed that people who ate their largest meal before 3 pm lost more weight.

2. Eat vegetables as a main course cooked in olive oil

I cannot stress this enough but this type of dish is the magic of the Greek diet. By eating a vegetable dish cooked in olive oil and tomato not only are you satisfied, but you are consuming 3-4 servings of vegetables in one sitting. These dishes are of moderate caloric level and low in carbs. Accompany it with a piece of feta cheese and you are set. Another benefit of eating vegetables as a main course is that because it is not a carb rich meal you will avoid the sleepiness that follows. For some Greek basic vegetables based main courses click here.

3. You should drink water mostly and sometimes tea, coffee and wine (for adults)

Yes, it is standard in some countries (like the US) to drink milk with meals, but is it really necessary? No. With the Mediterranean diet most dairy comes from cheese and yogurt, so save your calories and use them by eating solid food rather than liquid calories. The same goes for juice. Nobody really needs juice, eat your fruit. They are filling and you get all the fiber and nutrients. As for coffee and wine, each has its place in the

Mediterranean diet, but they do not replace water. Traditional Greek coffee has been associated with several health benefits and so has wine.

4. Consume the right amount of olive oil

More and more research is confirming what we here in the Mediterranean already know: good fat does not make you fat. Yes, calories count, but in order to sustain a vegetable based diet you need something to provide satiety and flavor; and that is olive oil. Olive oil not only makes all those vegetables delicious, it makes the meal filling. That does not mean, however, that you should be pouring olive oil mindlessly on everything. A good amount that is also associated with all the health benefits is about 3 tablespoons a day.

5. Move

The Mediterranean diet is not only a diet, it is a lifestyle, so moving around is imperative. Walking is fine, but general movement throughout the day is key. It's not enough to go to the gym for an hour in the morning and then sit at your office or on the couch the rest of the day. Take walking breaks, do some stretches every hour, do housework and if you can walk somewhere, do that instead of driving.

Printed in Great Britain
by Amazon